USING

QUERCETIN

FOR BEGINNERS

Unlocking The Health Benefits Of Quercetin, Potential Side Effects, Wellness Applications And More

DR. SPARKS RUBIO

DISCLAIMER

The information presented in this book is intended for general informational purposes only. It is not a substitute for professional medical advice, diagnosis, or treatment.

The author and publisher of this book have made every effort to ensure that the information provided is accurate and up-to-date at the time of publication. However, medical and scientific knowledge is constantly evolving, and new research may emerge. Therefore, the information in this book should not be considered a definitive source for medical or nutritional advice.

It is essential to consult with a qualified healthcare professional before making any decisions.

The author and publisher disclaim any liability for any adverse outcomes or consequences resulting from the use or misuse of the information in this book. Readers are urged to use their discretion and judgment when making decisions about their health and wellness.

By reading this book, you agree to do so at your own risk and should not use it as a substitute for professional medical advice or treatment.

TABLE OF CONTENTS

CHAPTER ONE

INTRODUCTION TO QUERCETIN

MEANING AND CLASSIFICATION

Plant pigment quercetin is a member of the flavonoid group, which is a broad category of phytonutrients. It is well known for both its numerous health advantages and strong antioxidant qualities. Quercetin belongs to the subclass of flavonoids called flavonols based on its chemical structure. Many plant-based foods have brilliant hues because flavonoids, which are plentiful in fruits, vegetables, and grains, are responsible for their color. Quercetin is unique among flavonoid cousins because of its exceptional bioactive capability and potential for medicinal use.

NATURAL QUERCETIN SOURCES

Quercetin is found naturally in a wide variety of fruits and vegetables. Apples, grapes, berries, onions, citrus fruits, cherries, and leafy green vegetables like spinach and kale are frequent foods that contain them. It is also present in significant levels in a variety of grains, seeds, and nuts. Because there are many different sources of quercetin, it can be incorporated into a variety of dietary patterns to meet a wide range of dietary needs and culinary tastes.

IMPORTANCE IN HISTORY

Quercetin has long been known for its therapeutic qualities and has been used in traditional medicine by many civilizations. Because of its anti-inflammatory, anti-allergic, and anti-carcinogenic qualities, it has been used for generations. Certain foods high in quercetin were prized for their therapeutic and illness-preventive properties in ancient cultures. The fact that quercetin has historical relevance confirms its continued value as a natural resource for enhancing health and well-being.

RELEVANCE AS A SUPPLEMENT TO A DIET

The value of quercetin as a dietary supplement has become increasingly well-known in modern times. Its ability to boost immunity, lower inflammation, and fight oxidative stress has made it a well-liked ingredient in nutritional supplements. The demand for quercetin as a dietary supplement has increased as people place a higher value on holistic approaches to wellness. Furthermore, studies are still revealing how effective it may be in reducing the risk of chronic illnesses like heart problems and some types of cancer. Thus, the acknowledgment of quercetin as a beneficial dietary supplement highlights its increasing importance in contemporary healthcare procedures and the wider wellness sector.

CHAPTER TWO

THE QUERCETIN SCIENCE

CHEMICAL COMPOSITION AND CHARACTERISTICS

One flavonoid that is present in many fruits, vegetables, and grains is quercetin, which is known to provide several health benefits. Its molecular structure is made up of a double bond on the carbon ring and a flavonol backbone with five hydroxyl groups. Because of this structure, quercetin possesses potent antioxidant qualities that enable it to scavenge free radicals, maintain cell membrane stability, and prevent damage caused by oxidative stress. Its overall antioxidative capability is also influenced by its ability to bind metal ions. Because of its diverse physiological effects, quercetin's molecular structure and functional groups make it a promising candidate for health advantages.

HOW THE BODY REACTS TO QUERCETIN

Quercetin functions in the human body via several different methods. As an antioxidant, it prevents oxidative damage to cells by scavenging free radicals and lowering the rate at which other molecules oxidize. Moreover, quercetin modifies gene expression and signaling pathways, which can affect several cellular functions such as apoptosis, proliferation, and inflammation. It has been noted to inhibit some important enzymes involved in inflammatory responses, including phospholipase and kinases. Furthermore, it has been discovered that quercetin affects the expression of multiple genes linked to the onset and spread of cancer, indicating a possible role for the supplement in the prevention and treatment of cancer.

THE CAPACITY TO ABSORB AND AVAIL

The effectiveness of quercetin in improving health is dependent on its bioavailability and absorption. Although quercetin can be found in a wide variety of plant-based foods, its chemical structure, dietary sources, and interactions with other nutrients can all affect how bioavailable it is. Studies indicate that consuming quercetin with specific meals or in combination with other flavonoids may enhance its absorption. Furthermore, certain gut microbes can increase its bioavailability by metabolizing quercetin into forms that are easier to absorb. Food preparation, for example, can degrade quercetin and lower its bioavailability, which could impede its absorption.

POSSIBLE HEALTH ADVANTAGES

The possible health advantages of quercetin have drawn interest from a variety of physiological systems. Due to its anti-inflammatory qualities, it may be able to help with inflammatory diseases like arthritis and several allergies. Additionally, by lowering the risk of atherosclerosis and enhancing heart function, quercetin's antioxidant ability may benefit cardiovascular health. By shielding neurons from oxidative stress and lowering neuroinflammation, studies also point to its promise in the fight against neurodegenerative disorders. Its potential to stop the proliferation of cancer cells and trigger apoptosis has also raised curiosity regarding its anticancer qualities. Research has also been done on quercetin's potential to improve immune function; studies have shown that it can strengthen the immune system and stimulate the immunological response.

All things considered, quercetin's varied characteristics and range of modes of action make it an intriguing natural substance with prospective uses in enhancing human health and averting several chronic illnesses. Its complete therapeutic potential will remain unclear unless more study is done on its bioavailability, modes of action, and distinct physiological effects. This research will also help guide its use in clinical settings.

QUINCETIN AND WELL-BEING

Because of its many health and wellness benefits, quercetin, a flavonoid found in a wide range of fruits, vegetables, and grains, has attracted a lot of attention. Its strong antioxidant qualities are one of its primary characteristics. Quercetin functions as a scavenger of dangerous free radicals and is essential for counteracting oxidative stress, which is linked to the development of several chronic illnesses, including cancer, neurological disorders, and cardiovascular diseases. Quercetin helps preserve cellular integrity and function by halting the oxidation of crucial components including proteins and lipids.

Additionally, quercetin plays a proactive role in the regulation of oxidative stress, a process linked to the onset of several diseases and the aging process. Through the regulation of specific enzyme activities and oxidative stress pathways, quercetin aids in maintaining the delicate equilibrium between the body's pro-oxidant and antioxidant processes. Using this mechanism, quercetin provides a shielding effect on cells, prolonging their life and averting early cellular deterioration and death.

KEEPING CELLS SAFE FROM DAMAGE

Its capacity to protect cells is further enhanced by its anti-inflammatory properties. It has been demonstrated that quercetin inhibits some inflammatory pathways and lowers the synthesis of inflammatory mediators, which lessens tissue damage brought on by inflammation. Quercetin can reduce the negative effects of chronic inflammation, which is becoming more widely acknowledged as a major factor in the pathophysiology of many chronic diseases, including diabetes, cardiovascular disorders, and arthritis. It does this by modifying the expression of different inflammatory genes and molecules.

Regarding its influence on the immune system, quercetin exhibits encouraging potential for augmenting the general function of the immune system. Through inducing immune cell activity, including T cells, B cells, and macrophages, quercetin enhances the body's defensive system against foreign invaders and diseases. This immune response enhancement is particularly important when it comes to fighting infections and stopping their spread, which in turn helps to lower the risk of contracting different diseases.

There has also been scientific interest in quercetin's potential to regulate immunological responses and allergies. According to studies, quercetin stabilizes mast cells and prevents histamine from being released, which is a major mediator of allergic reactions and may help reduce allergy symptoms. Furthermore, the immunomodulatory qualities of quercetin aid in immune response regulation, maintaining the body's equilibrium and control over the body's reactivity to allergens and reducing the intensity of allergy symptoms.

Applications of quercetin as a complement to traditional medicines in the management of chronic diseases are being investigated more and more. Quercetin is a good option for integrative treatment strategies that aim to improve the symptoms and progression of numerous chronic illnesses due to its capacity to reduce oxidative stress, inflammation, and immunological dysfunction.

CHAPTER THREE

HEART-RELATED HEALTH

HANDLING HEART CONDITIONS

Maintaining heart health is essential for longevity and general well-being. It entails a comprehensive strategy that incorporates several lifestyle adjustments, such as consistent exercise, a healthy diet, stress reduction, and abstaining from dangerous behaviors like smoking and binge drinking. Regular physical activity, such as aerobic workouts, enhances circulation, helps maintain healthy blood pressure levels, and strengthens the heart muscle.

Maintaining heart health also requires cutting back on processed carbohydrates and saturated fats while consuming a diet high in fruits, vegetables, healthy grains, and lean meats.

EFFECT ON CHOLESTEROL AND BLOOD PRESSURE

Essential functions of blood pressure and cholesterol are related to cardiovascular health. Hypertension, or high blood pressure, raises the risk of heart disease and stroke by putting undue strain on the heart and blood arteries. Reducing sodium intake, keeping a healthy weight, and engaging in regular physical activity are a few examples of lifestyle changes that can successfully lower blood pressure. Comparably, controlling cholesterol levels with a diet low in trans and saturated fats and high in good fats, such as those in nuts and avocados, can dramatically lessen the risk of artery plaque accumulation and heart disease.

METABOLIC WELL-BEING

Since metabolic conditions like diabetes and obesity can greatly raise the risk of developing cardiovascular diseases, the concepts of metabolic health and cardiovascular health are intimately related. A well-balanced and nutrient-dense diet, consistent exercise, and weight control are essential components of metabolic health management. Furthermore, maintaining adherence to prescribed drug regimens and insulin therapy for those with diabetes, as well as routine blood glucose testing, are critical in minimizing issues associated with cardiovascular health.

QUERCETIN AND THE CONTROL OF BLOOD SUGAR

The flavonoid quercetin, which may be found in a variety of fruits and vegetables like onions, berries, and apples, has drawn interest due to its possible function in controlling blood sugar levels. According to studies, quercetin may reduce blood glucose levels by blocking specific enzymes that are necessary for the metabolism of carbohydrates. Furthermore, it exhibits antioxidant qualities that may shield blood vessels from oxidative stress-caused damage, lowering the risk of cardiovascular issues linked to diabetes. Foods high in quercetin may help regulate blood sugar and improve cardiovascular health in general, but further research is required to determine its exact mechanism of action and therapeutic potential.

OBESITY AND WEIGHT MANAGEMENT

Due to its association with the development of hypertension, diabetes, and dyslipidemia, obesity is a major risk factor for cardiovascular disease. The prevention and management of obesity-related cardiovascular problems depend heavily on effective weight management techniques, which include a combination of nutritious eating practices and consistent physical exercise. This entails cutting back on processed and high-calorie meals, eating a balanced diet that emphasizes nutrient-dense foods, and controlling portion sizes to create a calorie deficit. A workout regimen that incorporates both aerobic and strength training can also help burn extra fat, increase muscle mass, and enhance cardiovascular fitness in general. Frequent assessment of body mass index (BMI) and weight can be useful markers of general cardiovascular health and advancements in weight control.

CHAPTER FOUR

QUERCETIN SUPPLEMENT

FOOD-BASED SOURCES

Plants contain quercetin, a flavonoid that is becoming more and more popular due to its possible health advantages. Although it can be acquired through diet, some people choose to take supplements of quercetin to fulfill their daily needs. Numerous fruits and vegetables, such as kale, apples, berries, onions, and citrus fruits, are excellent dietary sources of quercetin. These meals' vivid hue is often a reflection of the pigment that contains quercetin.

When compared to other vegetables, red onions in particular are recognized for having a comparatively high quercetin concentration. In a similar vein, apples especially their skin have high concentrations of this flavonoid. Including these foods high in quercetin in one's diet can provide a natural way to consume it.

VEGETABLES HIGH IN QUERCETIN

Some foods are particularly excellent sources of quercetin for people looking to up their consumption. Berries with vibrant colors, such as elderberries, blueberries, and cranberries, are a good source of quercetin and can be included in a well-balanced diet. Furthermore, this flavonoid is present in substantial concentrations in leafy greens like spinach and kale as well as veggies like broccoli. Fruits high in citrus, such as oranges, lemons, grapes, and cherries, add to the total amount of quercetin in the diet. People can increase their intake of quercetin naturally and possibly reap the benefits of its antioxidant qualities and other health-promoting effects by incorporating these foods into their regular diets.

RECOMMENDED CONSUMPTION OF FOOD

As there is no official necessary Dietary Allowance (RDA) for quercetin, it is not regarded as an essential nutrient, so the necessary dietary intake has not been determined with certainty. However, a general recommendation states that most people can safely consume up to 500 mg per day. This can be accomplished by eating a balanced diet that is high in foods high in quercetin. It is crucial to remember that each person's needs may differ depending on their age, sex, general health, and particular health objectives. Speaking with a medical expert can offer tailored advice on the right amount of quercetin to take depending on particular needs and circumstances.

DIFFERENT QUERCETIN SUPPLEMENT TYPES

Supplements containing quercetin have grown in popularity, especially among people who want to conveniently and carefully increase their levels of this flavonoid. Because these supplements come in a variety of formats, such as powders, tablets, and capsules, customers may simply obtain them. Additionally, some supplements combine quercetin with other bioactive ingredients, which may increase their overall health benefits. To guarantee product safety and performance, it is crucial to select a reliable brand of quercetin supplement that complies with quality standards and good production processes.

RECOMMENDED DOSAGE

The recommended dosage for supplements containing quercetin may change based on the particular product and its content. When taking quercetin supplements, the usual daily dosage is between 500 and 1000 mg, split into many doses. It is imperative, therefore, to adhere to the dosage guidelines supplied by the manufacturer or as advised by a medical expert. Without appropriate medical supervision, people should refrain from taking more than the recommended dosage because doing so could have unfavorable consequences or interact with other drugs or supplements.

POSSIBLE ADVERSE REACTIONS AND CONCURRENT EVENTS

When used in the recommended dosages, quercetin is usually thought to be safe for the majority of people. However, some people may have mild adverse effects, such as headaches, nausea, or upset stomach. Furthermore, quercetin may interfere with other medications, including blood thinners, antibiotics, and medications that the liver metabolizes. Therefore, before beginning a quercetin supplement program, people who are on any drugs or who already have health issues should speak with a healthcare provider. Before adding quercetin supplements to their daily routine, women who are pregnant or nursing should also consult a doctor to confirm that it is safe for the health of both the mother and the fetus.

CHAPTER FIVE

SELECTING AN APPROPRIATE QUERCETIN SUPPLEMENT

ASSESSMENT OF PRODUCT EXCELLENCE

To make sure the selected product is safe and effective, several criteria should be taken into account while assessing the quality of a quercetin supplement. The purity of quercetin itself is one of the most important things to evaluate. It is important to choose a supplement that only includes pure quercetin and doesn't include any artificial components, fillers, or needless additives. Third-party testing and certification are examples of quality control methods that can guarantee the supplement's effectiveness and purity. Among these certifications may be Good Manufacturing Practice (GMP) certifications, which attest to the fact that the product is produced in an establishment that satisfies exacting quality requirements.

Examining the Quercetin supplement's bioavailability is very crucial. The percentage of the swallowed dose that enters the systemic circulation is referred to as bioavailability. Poor bioavailability in certain supplements can lead to restricted absorption and decreased effectiveness. Selecting a supplement that employs methods like micronization or combining quercetin with components that promote absorption can assist in increasing the compound's bioavailability, guaranteeing that the body can absorb and use it efficiently.

WELL-KNOWN PRODUCTS AND BRANDS

When choosing a premium Quercetin supplement, brand reputation is also a crucial factor to take into account. Choosing goods from respectable, well-known brands can give another degree of security because these businesses are more likely to place a high priority on quality control and follow rigid manufacturing guidelines. Examining client testimonials and consulting medical experts for advice might provide important information about the safety and effectiveness of different quercetin supplements.

There are several well-known brands and goods on the market, all of which have unique formulas and extra components to enhance the possible health advantages of quercetin. Well-known companies in the dietary supplement market, including Nature's Way, NOW Foods, and Life Extension, provide supplements containing quercetin, which is well-known for its effectiveness and good quality. These companies frequently supply a wide range of quercetin products, such as pills, powders, and capsules, to accommodate the demands and preferences of various customers.

QUERCETIN MIXTURES

To maximize their health-promoting benefits, a lot of quercetin supplements are also made with complementing substances. Frequently, vitamin C is added to combos because it works in concert with quercetin to strengthen the immune system and function as a strong antioxidant. The natural enzyme bromelain, which is present in pineapple, when combined with quercetin can improve its anti-inflammatory and absorption qualities. In addition, certain supplements might include additional flavonoids or herbal extracts to produce all-encompassing formulas with a wider range of health advantages.

It's crucial to evaluate the scientific justification for adding other substances and their possible synergistic effects with quercetin when thinking about combinations containing quercetin.

CHAPTER SIX

USEFUL APPLICATIONS

ALLERGIES AND QUERCETIN

The natural plant pigment quercetin, sometimes referred to as a flavonoid, has attracted a lot of interest due to its possible advantages in the treatment of allergic reactions. Studies indicate that quercetin is an effective natural ingredient for reducing symptoms related to a variety of allergies because it has anti-inflammatory and antihistamine qualities. According to studies, quercetin may lessen the intensity of allergic reactions by preventing the body from releasing histamines and other inflammatory molecules. For those who are prone to allergic reactions, quercetin has demonstrated promise in reducing symptoms including congestion, itching, and sneezing by regulating the immune system's reactivity.

CONTROLLING ALLERGY RESPONSES

For people who are sensitive to certain allergens and environmental triggers, it is essential to effectively manage allergic reactions. Adding quercetin to allergy management regimens in addition to traditional medications has demonstrated the potential to offer further relief. Because quercetin stabilizes mast cells and prevents histamine from being released, it may help lessen the severity of allergic reactions. It's vital to remember that, even while quercetin could be helpful, it shouldn't be used as a stand-alone remedy. Instead, seeking advice from a medical expert is essential for thorough allergy control.

QUERCETIN AND SEASONAL ALLERGIES

The quality of life can be greatly affected by seasonal allergies, especially when there is an increased exposure to allergens. There has been interest in quercetin's potential to manage seasonal allergies; studies have suggested that its anti-inflammatory qualities may help reduce symptoms of seasonal allergic rhinitis. Quercetin may help alleviate symptoms of seasonal allergies, including watery, itchy eyes, sneezing, and nasal congestion, by regulating the immune system and lowering the release of inflammatory mediators. People looking for alternate ways to treat the symptoms of seasonal allergies have also been drawn to it because of its natural origin.

QUERCETIN FOR SPORTS PEOPLE

Maintaining optimal performance and reducing the physical effects of intense training are critical for athletes. Because it may improve physical performance and endurance, quercetin has gained attention as a possible supplement for sports. Quercetin may boost exercise capacity and mitochondrial biogenesis, according to certain research, which could result in improved athletic performance.

Through its ability to regulate energy production and lower oxidative stress, quercetin has the potential to enhance endurance and stamina, especially while engaging in prolonged physical activity.

ENHANCING ATHLETIC PERFORMANCE

Enhancing athletic performance can be achieved by a variety of tactics, such as diet and exercise plans. Because quercetin can increase the number of mitochondria in muscle cells and improve oxygen use, it may have a role in improving athletic performance. These mechanisms imply that supplementing with quercetin may result in enhanced aerobic capacity and a postponed onset of tiredness, allowing athletes to push their physical boundaries and provide their best during training and competition.

REST AND ACHES IN THE MUSCLES

In the context of sports rehabilitation, controlling muscular aches and encouraging effective healing are critical elements in maintaining peak performance. Research on quercetin's anti-inflammatory characteristics has focused on how it can help with muscle rehabilitation after exercise. Quercetin has the potential to expedite muscle recovery and mitigate pain in the muscles caused by exercise by mitigating inflammation and oxidative stress. Furthermore, quercetin may be useful in accelerating recovery, allowing athletes to restart training more successfully and minimize recovery time related to muscular soreness and exhaustion. This is because it can modify cellular signaling pathways involved in muscle regeneration.

QUERCETIN FOR HEALTHY SKIN

Quercetin is a flavonoid generated from plants that can be found in a variety of fruits, vegetables, and grains. It has gained interest due to its possible role in supporting healthy skin. As a powerful antioxidant and anti-inflammatory, quercetin is thought to provide several benefits when added to skincare regimens. It is a promising element in skincare due to its capacity to scavenge free radicals, suppress oxidative stress, and control inflammatory pathways. Quercetin can protect the skin from environmental aggressors and aid in its natural healing processes, which can help with a variety of skin issues and improve the health of the skin as a whole.

APPLICATIONS AND ADVANTAGES OF SKIN

Strong antioxidant capabilities are one of quercetin's main advantages for skin health. Quercetin helps to preserve collagen and elastin, two vital proteins that keep skin firm and supple, by scavenging free radicals, which can cause premature aging and skin damage. Consequently, this could help minimize the visibility of wrinkles, fine lines, and other age indicators, eventually promoting a more radiant and youthful complexion. Additionally, by reducing environmental damage brought on by pollution and UV radiation, its capacity to counteract oxidative stress may also aid in shielding the skin from possible harm.

Beyond its antioxidant capabilities, quercetin has also been shown to have anti-inflammatory properties. These properties can be especially helpful for people with inflammatory skin diseases like rosacea, eczema, or acne. Quercetin may help reduce redness, swelling, and irritation by modulating several inflammatory pathways, which may help to promote a more even-toned and balanced complexion. It can improve skin health and comfort overall by relieving irritated skin and lowering the intensity of inflammatory responses, which makes it an invaluable tool in the treatment of a variety of dermatological issues.

QUERCETIN COSMETICS

Quercetin is a substance that is found in a wide range of skincare products, such as lotions, masks, and serums. Quercetin-enriched formulas are frequently made to target certain skin conditions, providing a multidimensional approach to problems like UV damage, uneven skin tone, and hyperpigmentation. Quercetin is commonly used in anti-aging treatments because of its capacity to fight against photoaging and enhance the synthesis of collagen. This helps to restore the texture and tone of youthful skin. Its ability to reduce inflammation and improve overall skin resilience is further demonstrated by the fact that it is a component of treatments designed for skin types that are reactive or sensitive.

To maximize its effectiveness and provide all-encompassing skin benefits, quercetin is frequently combined with other synergistic substances including vitamin C, retinol, and hyaluronic acid as a component in skincare products.

By working together, we can maximize quercetin's anti-aging and antioxidant benefits while maintaining its best absorption and compatibility with other active components. With its adaptability and many advantages, quercetin keeps making a name for itself in the skincare sector by providing a safe, all-natural way for people to keep their skin looking young and healthy.

CHAPTER SEVEN

PROSPECTIVE STUDIES AND ADVANCEMENTS

CURRENT INVESTIGATIONS AND STUDIES

Many disciplines are currently working on continuing studies that have a lot of potential for the future in the current research landscape. In the realm of biotechnology, for example, scientists are exploring the complex workings of genetic engineering to unlock the possibilities of customized therapies and personalized medicine. Particularly, the study of CRISPR-Cas9 technology has drawn a lot of interest since it offers a novel approach to precise gene editing, which could completely change how genetic illnesses and inherited diseases are treated.

Concurrently, environmental science is placing more and more focus on creating long-term solutions to counteract climate change and its negative impacts. Scholars are delving into substitute energy sources, including sophisticated solar technology, biofuels, and innovative methods for capturing and storing carbon emissions. Innovative methods for reducing the environmental impact of human activity have been developed as a result of the integration of interdisciplinary study in disciplines such as ecology, engineering, and atmospheric science, paving the way for a more sustainable future for the earth.

PROSPECTIVE FIELDS OF STUDY

There is a great deal of promise for groundbreaking discoveries in several newly discovered scientific fields. For example, scientific study in the field of neuroscience is progressing quickly, aiming to decipher the workings of the human brain. Advances in neuroimaging techniques and state-of-the-art technologies like functional magnetic resonance imaging (fMRI) are helping scientists gain a better understanding of how the brain works, which will help in the development of more effective treatments for mental illnesses and neurological disorders.

In addition, the fields of machine learning and artificial intelligence (AI) are always developing, creating new opportunities for data analysis, automation, and improving decision-making processes in a variety of businesses. Researchers are investigating how AI might be integrated with a variety of industries, including finance, healthcare, and autonomous systems, to streamline processes, maximize resource use, and enhance overall effectiveness. There is still a great deal of interest in and research being done on the possible effects of AI in transforming several economic sectors.

PROSPECTIVE FUTURE FINDINGS

In the future, the combination of medicine and nanotechnology could lead to ground-breaking breakthroughs in the field of healthcare. The development of targeted drug delivery systems and nanoscale devices is anticipated by researchers, as these advancements potentially transform the diagnosis and treatment of diseases at the cellular level. The combination of biomedicine with nanotechnology presents a promising frontier in the fight against complicated diseases, such as cancer and other chronic illnesses, by offering the possibility of precise and least intrusive medicinal interventions.

In addition, as scientists work to use quantum mechanics to transform data encryption and information processing, the field of quantum computing is becoming more and more popular. Drug development, material science, and encryption could all be profoundly impacted by the development of quantum computers, which would have exponentially greater computational power. When practical quantum computing becomes a reality, it could revolutionize science and technology by providing solutions to intricate computational problems that are currently unsolvable by classical computers.

CONCLUSION

With more people becoming aware of quercetin's potential health advantages and exploring its many applications, the supplement's future looks bright. Quercetin is a flavonoid that may be found in many different fruits, vegetables, and grains. It has drawn interest because of its potential to improve general health and well-being as well as its supposed anti-inflammatory and antioxidant qualities.

The scientific community has been working harder in recent years to determine whether quercetin may be used as a therapy to treat and prevent a variety of illnesses. Its ability to fight chronic illnesses such as cancer, neurological disorders, and cardiovascular problems has made it a substance of great interest in the field of preventive medicine.

Furthermore, there has been interest in quercetin's purported ability to enhance immunity, especially given the current global health issues that highlight the significance of bolstering the body's defense mechanisms. Given its supposed antiviral and antibacterial qualities and its potential as a natural immune modulator, more research into this area seems highly promising, particularly in light of the rise in infectious disorders and antibiotic resistance.

In addition, the growing popularity of taking a more holistic approach to well-being and health has raised demand for natural supplements like quercetin. Quercetin's market potential as a dietary supplement is being propelled by consumers' increased desire for naturally produced products and their increasing search for alternatives to synthetic substances.

The continuous progress in technology and formulation methodologies has additionally enabled the creation of inventive delivery strategies, augmenting Quercetin's bioavailability and effectiveness. For example, methods based on nanotechnology have demonstrated potential in enhancing quercetin's absorption and targeted distribution, thereby optimizing its therapeutic effects and reducing any related side effects.